CW00584706

Ketogenic Diet Cookbook

Find Success on the Ketogenic Diet with These Simple and Delicious Low-Carb, High-Fat Recipes

The Wellness Foodie

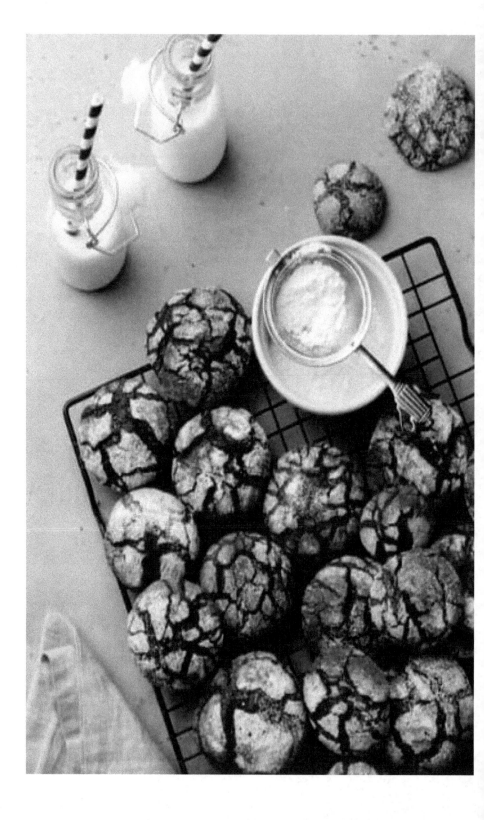

Table of Contents

© **Copyright 2020 by The Wellness Foodie - All rights reserved.**

The following Book is reproduced below with the goal of providing information that is as accurate and reliable as possible. Regardless, purchasing this Book can be seen as consent to the fact that both the publisher and the author of this book are in no way experts on the topics discussed within and that any recommendations or suggestions that are made herein are for entertainment purposes only. Professionals should be consulted as needed prior to undertaking any of the action endorsed herein.

This declaration is deemed fair and valid by both the American Bar Association and the Committee of Publishers Association and is legally binding throughout the United States.

Furthermore, the transmission, duplication, or reproduction of any of the following work including specific information will be considered an illegal act irrespective of if it is done electronically or in print. This extends to creating a secondary or tertiary copy of the work or a recorded copy and is only allowed with the express written consent from the Publisher. All additional right reserved.

The information in the following pages is broadly considered a truthful and accurate account of facts and as such, any inattention, use, or misuse of the information in question by the reader will render any resulting actions solely under their purview. There are no scenarios in which the publisher or the original author of this work can be in any fashion deemed liable for any hardship or damages that may befall them after undertaking information described herein.

Additionally, the information in the following pages is intended only for informational purposes and should thus be thought of as universal. As befitting its nature, it is presented without assurance regarding its prolonged validity or interim quality. Trademarks that are mentioned are done without written consent and can in no way be considered an endorsement from the trademark holder.

Introduction

Ketogenic Diet

"Ketogenic" is a term for a low-carb diet. You can get more calories from protein and fat and less from carbohydrates by following a ketogenic diet. A keto diet is especially useful for losing excess body fat, reducing hunger, and improving type-2 diabetes or metabolic syndrome.

A keto or ketogenic diet is a low-carb, adequate protein, higher-fat diet that can help you burn fat more effectively. It has many benefits for weight loss, health, and performance.

While you eat far fewer carbohydrates on a keto diet, you maintain adequate protein consumption and may increase your intake of fat. The reduction in the carb intake puts your body in a metabolic state called ketosis, where fat, from your diet, and from your body, is burned to make energy.

People use a ketogenic diet most often to lose weight, but it can also help manage certain medical conditions, like epilepsy, heart disease, certain brain diseases, and even acne. A ketogenic diet uses more calories to change fat into energy than it does to change carbs into energy. It reduces carbs that are easy to digest, like sugar, soda, pastries, and white bread.

A keto diet can result in a calmer stomach, less gas, fewer cramps and less pain. It can increase your physical endurance by improving your access to the vast amounts of energy in your fat stores.

When you suddenly switch your body's metabolism from burning carbs (glucose) to fat and ketones, you may have some side effects as your body gets used to its new fuel. During this period, symptoms may include headache, tiredness, muscle fatigue, cramping, and heart palpitations. These side effects are short-term for most people, and there are ways to minimize or cure them.

Benefits of a Ketogenic Diet

- Weight loss and maintenance
- Reduced carbohydrate consumption plays a role in reducing your appetite
- Improvement in the quality of sleep
- Higher energy levels
- Improves emotional disposition
- Improves heart health
- Improves liver health
- Improves cognition
- Controls blood sugar and may reverse type-2 diabetes

Ketogenic Diet Risks:

- Nutrient deficiency
- Liver problems
- Kidney problems
- Constipation
- Fuzzy thinking and mood swings

Foods Allowed in the Ketogenic Diet:

- Low-carb vegetables
- Shirataki noodles
- Unsweetened tea
- Butter and cream
- Seafood

- Eggs
- Cheese
- Avocados
- Meat and poultry
- Dark chocolate and cocoa powder
- Unsweetened coffee
- Nuts and seeds
- Berries
- Olives
- Coconut oil
- Plain Greek yogurt and cottage cheese

Foods Not Allowed in the Ketogenic Diet

- Honey, syrup, or sugar in any form
- Chips and crackers
- Baked goods, including gluten-free
- Corn
- Grains
- Juices
- Rice
- Potato and sweet potato
- Starchy vegetables and high-sugar fruits
- Sweetened yogurt

10 Day Meal Plan

Days	Breakfast	Lunch	Dinner
Day 1	Scrambled eggs in butter on a bed of lettuce topped with avocado	Spinach salad with grilled salmon	Pork chop with cauliflower mash and red cabbage slaw
Day 2	Bulletproof coffee (made with butter and coconut oil), hard-boiled eggs	Tuna salad in stuffed tomatoes	Meatballs on zucchini noodles, topped with cream sauce
Day 3	Cheese and veggie omelet topped with salsa	Sashimi takeout with miso soup	Roasted chicken with asparagus and sautéed mushrooms
Day 4	Smoothie made with almond milk, greens, almond butter, and protein powder	Chicken tenders made with almond flour with greens, goat cheese & cucumbers	Grilled shrimp topped with a lemon butter sauce with a side of asparagus
Day 5	Fried eggs with bacon and a side of greens	Grass-fed burger in a lettuce "bun" topped with avocado and a side salad	Baked tofu with cauliflower rice, broccoli, and peppers, topped with homemade peanut sauce
Day 6	Baked eggs in	Poached salmon	Grilled beef

		avocado rolls wrapped in seaweed (rice-free)	kebabs with peppers and sautéed broccolini
Day 7	Eggs scrambled with veggies, topped with salsa	Sardine salad made with mayo in half an avocado	Broiled trout with butter, sautéed bok choy
Day 8	Keto egg muffins	Lettuce wraps with BBQ chicken	Italian keto meatballs with mozzarella cheese
Day 9	Scrambled eggs in butter on a bed of lettuce topped with avocado	Keto chicken burger with jalapeno aioli	Crispy tuna burgers
Day 10	Cheese crusted omelet	Asian keto chicken stir-fry with broccoli	Tex-Mex stuffed zucchini boats

Breakfast

Minty Green Smoothie

Servings: 2

Preparation Time: 10 minutes

Per Serving: Net Carbs 4g Cal 293 Fat 15g Saturated Fat 2g
Carbs 11g Fiber 7g Protein 28g

Ingredients:

- 1 lb avocado
- 2 Cups fresh spinach
- 20 Drops of sweet leaf liquid stevia peppermint Sweet drops
- 2 Scoop whey protein powder
- 1 Cup unsweetened almond milk
- 1/2 Tsp peppermint extract
- 1 Cup ice
- Optional: Cacao nibs

Procedure:

1. Firstly, in a blender, place avocado, spinach, protein powder and milk and mix until smooth.
2. Then, add stevia Peppermint Sweet Drop Sweet Leaf Liquid, sugar, and ice, and blend until frosty.
3. Now, stevia can be tasted and adjusted as needed.

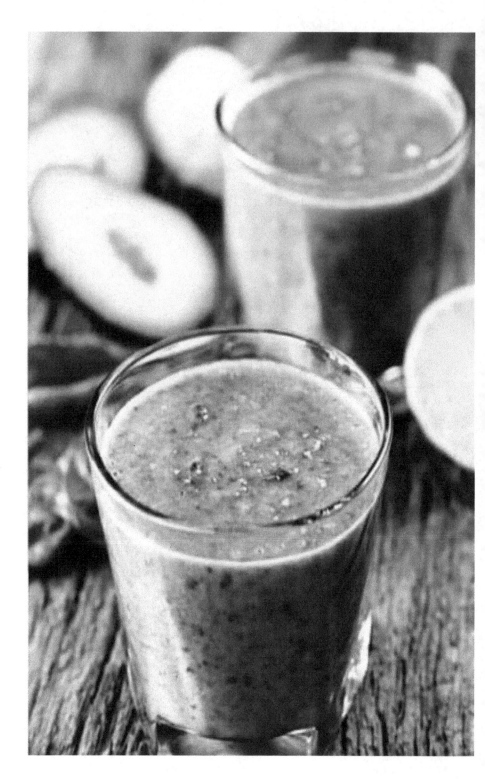

Tasty Green Smoothie

Servings: 10

Preparation Time: 5 minutes

Per Serving: 375 Cal, 25g Fat, 30g Protein, 4g Net Carbs

Ingredients:

- 2 Oz spinach
- 110 G cucumber
- 3 Cups almond milk
- 100 g celery
- 100 g avocado
- 2 Tbsp of coconut oil
- 20 Drops of stevia liquid
- 1 Scoop pure Protein Powder
- 1 Tsp chia seeds (to garnish).
- 1 Tsp matcha powder

Procedure:

1. First, place almond milk and spinach in a blender or nutria bullet.
2. Mix spinach for a few seconds to make room for the rest of the ingredients.

3. Then, add the remaining ingredients and mix for a minute until creamy.
4. Now, garnish with chia seeds in a dish.

Easy Tropical Pink Smoothie

Servings: 10

Preparation Time: 5 hours

Per Serving: Net carbs 12.1 g Protein 24.6 g Fat 28.6 g Cal 403

Ingredients:

- 1 Dragon fruit
- 2 Small wedge galia melon
- 1 Cup full-fat cream or coconut milk
- 2 Scoop of whey protein powder (vanilla or plain), white egg powder or hydrolyzed gelatin powder
- 2 Tbsp chia seeds
- 12 Drops Stevia extract oil
- 3 Cup water

Procedure:

Blend all ingredients until they are smooth.

Acai Almond Butter Smoothie

Servings: 8

Preparation Time: 5 minutes

Per Serving: Cal 345 Fat 20 Carbs 8 Fiber 2 Protein 15

Ingredients:

- 1 100g Pack unsweetened acai puree
- ¾ Cup unsweetened almond milk
- 1/8 Avocado
- 1.1/2 Tbsp collagen or protein powder
- 1/2 Tbsp coconut oil
- 1/2 Tbsp Almond Butter
- 1/4 Tsp vanilla extract
- 1 Drop liquid stevia (optional)

Procedure:

1. If you are using individualized 100-gram packs of acai puree, run the package under lukewarm water for a few seconds until you can break up the puree into small pieces.
2. Place it in the blender.
3. Then, add remaining ingredients and blend until smooth.
4. Add more water or ice cubes as needed.
5. Now, drizzle the almond butter to make it look beautiful on the side of the glass.

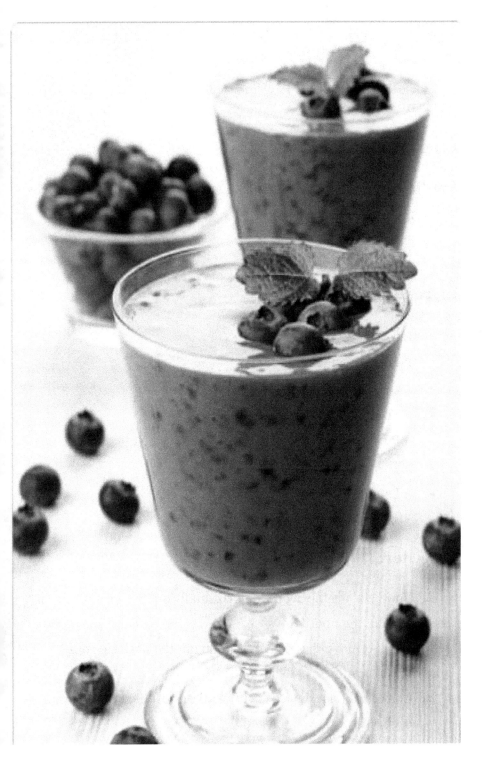

Delightful Avocado Bun Breakfast Burger

Servings: 4

Preparation Time: 15 minutes

Per Serving: -717 Cal, 61.36g Fat, 20.11g Carbs, 14.6g Fiber, 2.88g Sugar, 27.41g Protein

Ingredients:

- 2 Eggs
- 2 Tbsp. sesame seeds
- 2 Oz breakfast sausage
- 2 Tbsp mayonnaise
- 2 Pinch salt and pepper
- 2 Tbsp olive oil
- 2 Lettuce leaf

Procedure:

1. Firstly, place the avocado horizontally on its side and slice it right in the middle.
2. Then, remove the seed and spoon out the flesh carefully.
3. Heat the oil in a skillet.
4. Cook breakfast sausage over medium-low heat for 1-2 min on each side until well toasted.

5. In the skillet, crack the egg open, turn the heat down, cover and cook with the sunny side up. Make sure that the egg white is fully cooked.

6. Place the lower half of the avocado on a plate, spoon some mayo into the avocado hole and top with lettuce, tomato, sausage

7. Now, add the egg carefully and top with the other half of the avocado.

8. Sprinkle salt, pepper and sesame seeds as desired.

Delectable Keto Cheese Omelet

Servings: 4

Preparation Time: 15 minutes

Per Serving: Fat 80g, protein 40g, Net carbs 4g, Cal 897

Ingredients:

- 6 Oz butter
- 12 Eggs
- 14 Oz shredded cheddar cheese
- Salt and pepper to taste

Procedure:

1. First, mix the eggs smoothly, then blend in half of the cheddar.
2. Melt the butter in a hot frying pan, pour the egg mixture and leave for a few min
3. Then, reduce the heat and add the remaining shredded cheese.
4. Finally, fold the omelet and serve immediately.

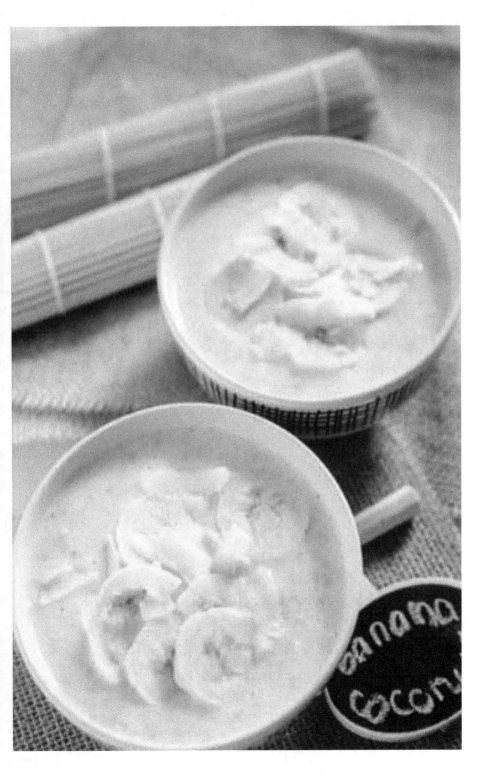

Coconut Porridge

Servings: 2

Preparation Time: 10 minutes

Per Serving: Fat 49g, Protein 9g, Net carbs 4g, Cal 486

Ingredients:

- 2 Egg, beaten
- 2 Tbsp coconut flour
- 2 Pinch salt
- 8 Tbsp coconut cream
- 2 Oz butter or coconut oil

Procedure:

1. Firstly, mix the egg, coconut flour and psyllium husk powder in a small bowl.
2. Melt the butter or coconut oil over low heat.
3. Then, slowly whisk the egg mixture to achieve a thick creamy texture.
4. Now, add fresh berries to your porridge and enjoy.
5. Finally, serve with coconut milk or cream.

No Bread Keto Breakfast Sandwich

Servings: 4

Preparation Time: 10 minutes

Per Serving: Fat 30g, Protein 20g, Net carbs 2g, Cal 354

. Ingredients:

- 8 Eggs
- 2 Oz smoked deli ham
- 4 Oz cheddar or Provolone cheese, cut in thick slices
- Salt and pepper
- Tabasco sauce

Procedure:

1. Firstly, heat butter frying pan over medium heat.
2. Then, fry the eggs on both sides and add salt and pepper.
3. For each "sandwich," use a fried egg as the base.
4. Place the ham on top, then add the cheese.
5. Use a fried egg to top off each stack.
6. Now, leave the cheese to melt over low heat if desired.
7. Finally, serve immediately with a few drops of Tabasco sauce.

Tasty Triple Cheese and Bacon Zucchini Balls

Servings: 12

Preparation Time: 30 minutes

Per Serving: calories: 406 | fat: 26.7g | protein: 33.3g | carbs: 8.6g | net carbs: 5.7g | fiber: 2.9g

Ingredients:

- 8 cups zucchini, spiralized
- 1 Pound (227 g) bacon, chopped
- 12 Ounces (170 g) cottage cheese, curds
- 12 Ounces (170 g) cream cheese
- 1 Cup fontina cheese
- 1 Cup dill pickles, chopped, squeezed
- 4 Cloves garlic, crushed
- 2 cups grated Parmesan cheese
- 1 teaspoon caraway seeds
- 1 Teaspoon dried dill weed
- 1 Teaspoon onion powder
- Salt and black pepper, to taste
- 2 cups crushed pork rinds
- Cooking oil

Procedure:

1. Firstly, thoroughly mix zoodles, cottage cheese, dill pickles, ½ cup of Parmesan cheese, garlic, cream cheese, bacon, and Fontina cheese until well combined.
2. Shape the mixture into balls.
3. Refrigerate for 3 hours.
4. Then, in a mixing bowl, mix the remaining ½ cup of Parmesan cheese, crushed pork rinds, dill, black pepper, onion powder, caraway seeds, and salt.
5. Roll cheese ball in Parmesan mixture to coat.
6. Now, set a skillet over medium heat and warm 1-inch of oil.
7. Fry cheeseballs until browned on all sides.
8. Finally, set on a paper towel to soak up any excess oil.

Yummy Mozzarella and Chorizo Omelet

Servings: 2

Preparation Time: 10 minutes

Per Serving: calories: 452 | fat: 36.4g | protein: 30.1g | carbs: 5.4g | net carbs: 2.9g | fiber: 2.5g

Ingredients:

- 4 Eggs
- 12 Basil leaves
- 4 Ounces (57 g) Mozzarella cheese
- 2 Tablespoons butter
- 2 Tablespoons water
- 8 Thin slices chorizo
- 1 Tomato, sliced
- Salt and black pepper, to taste

Procedure:

1. Firstly, whisk the eggs along with the water and some salt and pepper.
2. Melt the butter in a skillet and cook the eggs for 30 seconds.
3. Spread the chorizo slices over.
4. Then, arrange the tomato and Mozzarella over the chorizo.

5. Cook for about 3 minutes.

6. Now, cover the skillet and cook for 3 minutes until omelet is set.

7. When ready, remove the pan from heat; run a spatula around the edges of the omelet and flip it onto a warm plate, folded side down.

8. Finally, serve garnished with basil leaves and green salad.

Easy Bacon and Zucchini Hash

Servings: 2

Preparation Time: 25 minutes

Per Serving: calories: 341 | fat: 26.7g | protein: 17.3g | carbs: 7.3g | net carbs: 6.5g | fiber: 0.8g

Ingredients:

- 2 Mediums zucchini, diced
- 4 Bacon slices
- 2 Eggs
- 2 Tablespoons coconut oil
- 1 Small onion, chopped
- 2 Tablespoons chopped parsley
- 1/2 Teaspoon salt

Procedure:

1. Firstly, place the bacon in a skillet and cook for a few minutes, until crispy.
2. Remove and set aside.
3. Then, warm the coconut oil and cook the onion until soft, for about 3-4 minutes, occasionally stirring.

4. Now, add the zucchini, and cook for 10 more minutes until zucchini is brown and tender, but not mushy.
5. Finally, transfer to a plate and season with salt.
6. Crack the egg into the same skillet and fry over medium heat.
7. Top the zucchini mixture with the bacon slices and a fried egg.
8. Serve hot, sprinkled with parsley.

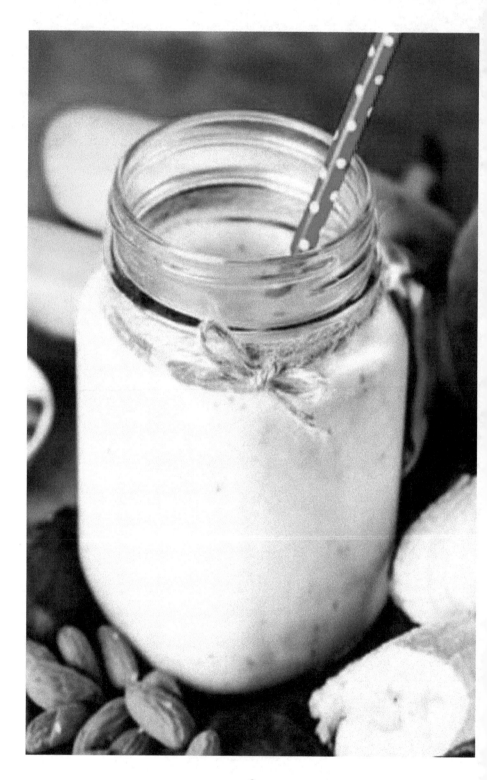

Delicious Almond Shake

Servings: 2

Preparation Time: 5 minutes

Per Serving: calories: 325 | fat: 26.9g | protein: 19.1g | carbs: 8.1g | net carbs: 6.0g | fiber: 2.1g

Ingredients:

- 3 Cups almond milk
- 4 Tablespoons almond butter ½ teaspoon almond extract
- 1 Teaspoon cinnamon
- 4 Tablespoons flax meal
- 1 Tablespoon collagen peptides
- A pinch of salt
- 30 Drops of stevia
- A handful of ice cubes

Procedure:

1. Firstly, add almond milk, almond butter, flax meal, almond extract, collagen peptides, a pinch of salt, and stevia to the bowl of a blender.
2. Blitz until uniform and smooth, for about 30 seconds.
3. Then, add a bit more almond milk if it's very thick.

4. Now, taste and adjust flavor as needed, adding more stevia for sweetness or almond butter to the creaminess.

5. Finally, pour in a smoothie glass, add the ice cubes and sprinkle with cinnamon.

Flavorful Cream Cheese Salmon Omelet Roll

Servings: 2

Preparation Time: 15 minutes

Per Serving: calories: 512 | fat: 47.8g | protein: 36.8g | carbs: 13.0g | net carbs: 5.7g | fiber: 7.3g

Ingredients:

- 1 Avocado, sliced
- 4 Tablespoons chopped chives
- 1 Package smoked salmon, cut into strips
- 2 Spring onions, sliced
- 6 Eggs
- 4 Tablespoons cream cheese
- 2 Tablespoons butter
- Salt and black pepper, to taste

Procedure:

1. Firstly, in a small bowl, combine the chives and cream cheese; set aside.
2. Beat the eggs in a large bowl and season with salt and black pepper.

3. Then, melt the butter in a pan over medium heat.
4. Add the eggs to the pan and cook for about 3 minutes.
5. Flip the omelet over and continue cooking for another 2 minutes until golden.
6. Now, remove the omelet to a plate and spread the chive mixture over.
7. Arrange the salmon, avocado, and onion slices.
8. Finally, wrap the omelet and serve immediately.

Lunch

Tasty Chicken and Broccoli Gratin

Servings: 4

Preparation Time: 20 minutes

Per Serving: Calories: 612 Fat: 48 g Carbs: 11 g Protein 34 g Sugar: 1 g

Ingredients:

- 2 Pound of chicken breasts
- 1/2 Cup almond butter
- 100 Cl of fresh cream
- 1 Cup goat cheese
- 4 Organic eggs
- 4 Crushed garlic cloves
- 2 Pinch of salt
- 2 Pinch of pepper

Procedure:

1. Firstly, cook the broccoli in a pot of water for 10 minutes. It must remain firm.
2. Melt the butter in a skillet; add the crushed garlic clove and the salted and peppered chicken.
3. Let it get a brown color.

4. Then, drain the broccoli and mix with the chicken.

5. Beat the eggs with the cream, salt, and pepper.

6. Place broccoli and chicken in a baking dish, cover with cream mixture and sprinkle with grated cheese.

7. Put in the oven at 390°F for 20 minutes.

8. When the gratin is ready; set it aside to cool for 3 minutes

9. Now, put the gratin into two halves or in four portions

10. Finally, place every two portions of gratin in a container so that you have two containers.

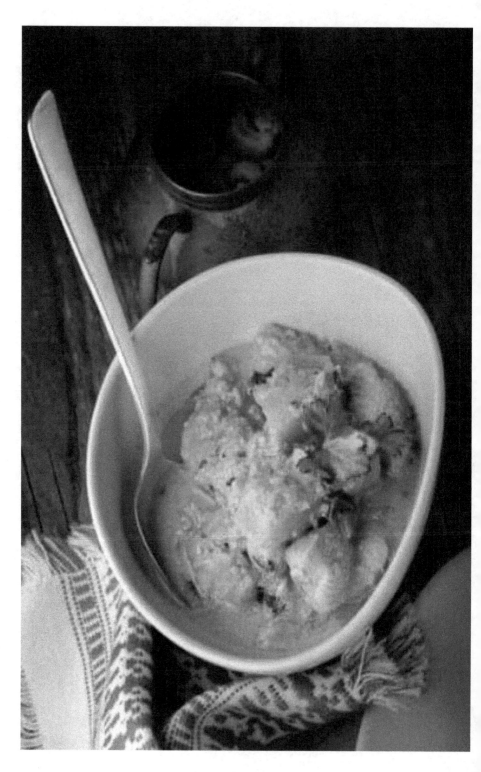

Chicken Curry

Servings: 4

Preparation Time: 40 minutes

Per Serving: 626 Fat: 53.2 g Carbs: 9 g Protein 27.8 g Sugar: 3 g;

Ingredients:

- 4 Chicken breasts
- 2 Garlic clove
- 1 Small onion
- 2 Zucchinis
- 2 Carrots
- 2 Box of bamboo shoots or sprouts
- 2 Cup coconut milk
- 2 Tbsp. tomato paste
- 4 Tbsp yellow curry paste

Procedure:

1. Firstly, mince the onion and sauté in a pan with a little oil for a few minutes.
2. Then, add chicken cut in large cubes and crushed garlic, salt, pepper and sauté quickly over high heat until meat begins to color.

3. Pour zucchini and carrots in thick slices into the pan.

4. Sear over high heat for a few minutes, then add the coconut milk, tomato sauce, bamboo shoots and one to two tbsps. curry paste, depending on your taste.

5. Now, cook over low heat and cover for 30 to 45 minutes, stirring occasionally

6. Once cooked, divide the chicken curry between 2 containers

7. Finally, store the containers in the refrigerator

Delicious Bacon Wrapped Asparagus

Servings: 4

Preparation Time: 30 minutes

Per Serving: Calories: 204 Carbs: 1.4g Protein: 5.9g Fat: 19.3g
Sugar: 0.5g

Ingredients:

- 1 cup heavy whipping cream
- 4 bacon slices, precooked
- 8 small spears asparagus
- Salt, to taste
- 2 tablespoon butter

Procedure:

1. Firstly, preheat the oven to 360 degrees and grease a baking sheet with butter.
2. Meanwhile, mix cream, asparagus and salt in a bowl.
3. Then, wrap the asparagus in bacon slices and arrange them in the baking dish.
4. Transfer the baking dish to the oven and bake for about 20 minutes.
5. Remove from the oven and serve hot.

6. Now, place the bacon wrapped asparagus in a plate and put aside to chill for meal prepping.
7. Split it in 2 containers and cover the lid.
8. Finally, refrigerate for about 2 days and reheat in the microwave before serving.

Tempting Spinach Chicken

Servings: 4

Preparation Time: 20 minutes

Per Serving: Calories: 288 Carbs: 3.6g Protein: 27.7g Fat: 18.3g
Sugar: 0.3g

Ingredients:

- 4 garlic cloves, minced
- 4 tablespoons unsalted butter, divided
- 1/2 cup parmesan cheese, shredded
- ¾ pound chicken tenders
- 1/2 cup heavy cream
- 20 ounces frozen spinach, chopped
- Salt and black pepper, to taste

Procedure:

1. Firstly, heat 1 tablespoon of butter in a large skillet and add chicken, salt and black pepper.
2. Cook for about 3 minutes on both sides and remove the chicken to a bowl.
3. Then, melt remaining butter in the skillet and add garlic, cheese, heavy cream and spinach.

4. Cook for about 2 minutes and add the chicken.

5. Cook for about 5 minutes on low heat and dish out to immediately serve.

6. Place chicken in a saucer and set apart to cool for meal prepping.

7. Split it in 2 containers and cover them.

8. Finally, refrigerate for about 3 days and reheat in microwave before serving.

Flavorful Lemon Grass Prawns

Servings: 4

Preparation Time: 25 minute

Per Serving: Calories: 322 Carbs: 3.8g Protein: 34.8g Fat: 18g
Sugar: 0.1g Sodium: 478mg

Ingredients:

- 1 red chili pepper, seeded and chopped
- 4 lemongrass stalks
- 1 pound prawns, deveined and peeled
- 12 tablespoons butter
- 1/2 teaspoon smoked paprika

Procedure:

1. Firstly, preheat the oven to 390 degrees and grease a baking dish.
2. Mix together red chili pepper, butter, smoked paprika and prawns in a bowl.
3. Then, marinate for about 2 hours and then thread the prawns on the lemongrass stalks.
4. Arrange the threaded prawns on the baking dish and transfer it in the oven.
5. Now, bake for about 15 minutes and dish out to serve immediately.

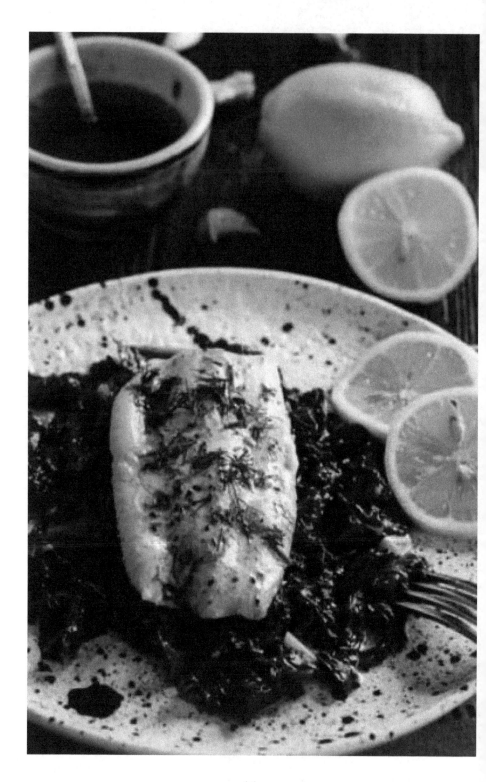

Salmon Stew

Servings: 4

Preparation Time: 20 minutes

Per Serving: Calories: 272 Carbs: 4.4g Protein: 32.1g Fat: 14.2g Sugar: 1.9g

Ingredient:

- 2-pounds salmon fillet, sliced
- 2 onions, chopped
- Salt, to taste
- 1 tablespoon butter, melted
- 2 cups fish broth
- 1 teaspoon red chili powder

Procedure:

1. Firstly, season the salmon fillets with salt and red chili powder.
2. Put butter and onions in a skillet and sauté for about 3 minutes.
3. Add seasoned salmon and cook for about 2 minutes on each side.
4. Then, add fish broth and secure the lid.
5. Cook for about 7 minutes on medium heat and open the lid.
6. Dish out and serve immediately.

7. Now, transfer the stew in a bowl and set aside to cool for meal prepping. 8.

8. Divide the mixture into 2 containers.

9. Cover the containers and

10. Refrigerate for about 2 days. Reheat in the microwave before

Enjoyable Asparagus Salmon Fillets

Servings: 4

Preparation Time: 30 minutes

Per Serving: 475 Carbs: 1.1g Protein: 35.2g Fat: 36.8g Sugar: 0.5g
Sodium: 242mg

Ingredients:

- 2 teaspoons olive oil
- 8 asparagus stalks
- 4 salmon fillets
- 1/2 cup butter
- 1/2 cup champagne
- Salt and freshly ground black

Procedure:

1. Firstly, preheat the oven to 355 degrees and grease a baking dish.
2. Put all the ingredients in a bowl and mix well.
3. Then, put this mixture in the baking dish and transfer it to the oven.
4. Bake for about 20 minutes and dish out.

5. Place the salmon fillets in a dish and set aside to cool for meal prepping.
6. Divide it into 2 containers and close the lid.
7. Now, refrigerate for 1 day and reheat in microwave before serving.

Pleasant Crispy Baked Chicken

Servings: 4

Preparation Time: 40 minutes

Per Serving: Calories: 304 Carbs: 1.4g Protein: 26.1g Fat: 21.6g
Sugar: 0.1g Sodium: 137mg

Ingredients:

- 4 tablespoons butter
- 1/2 teaspoon turmeric powder
- 1/2 cup sour cream
- Salt and black pepper, to taste

Procedure:

1. Firstly, preheat the oven to 360 degrees and grease a baking dish with butter.
2. Season the chicken with turmeric powder, salt and black pepper in a bowl.
3. Then, put the chicken on the baking dish and transfer it to the oven.
4. Bake for about 10 minutes and dish out to serve topped with sour cream.

5. Now, transfer the chicken in a bowl and set aside to cool for meal prepping.
6. Divide it into 2 containers and cover the containers.
7. Finally, refrigerate for up to 2 days and reheat in microwave before serving.

Flavorful Sour and Sweet Fish

Servings: 4

Preparation Time: 25 minutes

Per Serving: Calories: 258 Carbs: 2.8g Protein: 24.5g Fat: 16.7g
Sugar: 2.7g Sodium: 649mg

Ingredients:

- 4 drops stevia
- 1/2 cup butter, melted
- Salt and black pepper, to taste

Procedure:

1. Firstly, put butter and fish chunks in a skillet and cook for about 3 minutes.
2. Then, add stevia salt and black pepper and cook for about 10 minutes,
3. Stirring continuously.
4. Dish out in a bowl and serve immediately.
5. Now, place fish in a dish and put aside to chill for meal prepping.
6. Separate it in 2 containers and refrigerate for up to 2 days.
7. Finally, preheat in microwave before serving.

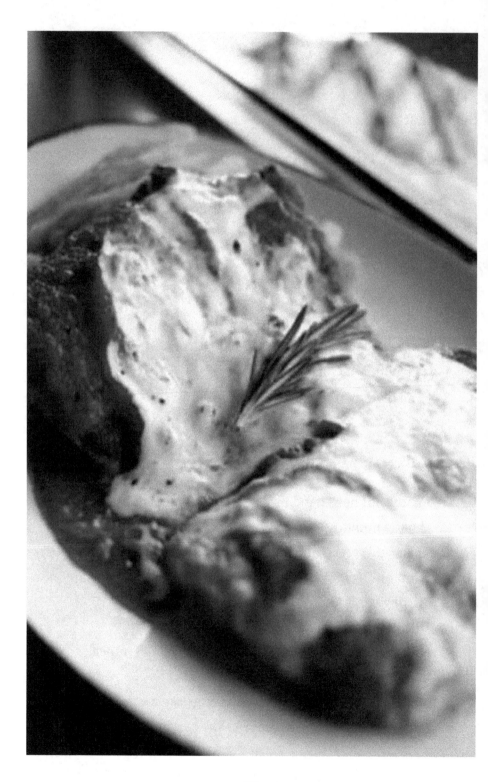

Delectable Creamy Chicken

Servings: 4

Preparation Time: 25 minutes

Per Serving: Calories: 335 Carbs: 2.9g Protein: 34g Fat: 20.2g
Sugar: 0.8g Sodium: 154mg

Ingredients:

- 1/2 cup sour cream
- 1/2 cup mushrooms
- 1 small onion, chopped
- 2 tablespoons butter
- 1 pound chicken breasts

Procedure:

1. First, heat butter in a skillet and add onions and mushrooms.
2. Sauté for about 5 minutes and add chicken breasts and salt.
3. Secure the lid and cook for about 5 more minutes.
4. Then, add sour cream and cook for about 3 minutes.
5. Open the lid and dish out in a bowl to serve immediately.
6. Now, transfer the creamy chicken breasts in a dish and set aside to cool for meal prepping.
7. Divide them in 2 containers and cover their lid.
8. Finally, refrigerate for 2-3 days and reheat in microwave before serving.

Rice Wine Duck with White Onion

Servings: 12

Preparation Time: 30 minutes

Per Serving: 264 | fat: 11.4g | protein: 34.2g | carbs: 3.6g | net carbs: 3.0g | fiber: 0.6g

Ingredients:

- 3 pounds (680 g) duck breast 1 tablespoon sesame oil
- 2 white onions, chopped
- 1/2 cup rice wine
- 6 teaspoons soy sauce

Procedure:

1. Firstly, gently score the duck breast skin in a tight crosshatch pattern using a sharp knife.
2. Heat the sesame oil in a skillet over moderate heat.
3. Now, sauté the onion until tender and translucent.
4. Then, add in the duck breasts; sear the duck breasts for 10 to 13 minutes or until the skin looks crispy with golden brown color; drain off the duck fat from the skillet.
5. Flip the breasts over and sear the other side for 3 minutes.

6. Deglaze the skillet with rice wine, scraping up any brown bits stuck to the bottom.

7. Transfer to a baking pan; add the rice wine and soy sauce to the baking pan.

8. Now, roast in the preheated oven at 400°F (205°C) for 4 minutes for medium-rare (145°F / 63°C), or 6 minutes for medium (165°F / 74°C).

9. Finally, serve garnished with sesame seeds if desired. Enjoy!

Yummy Chicken Puttanesca

Servings: 10

Preparation Time: 35 minutes

Per Serving: calories: 266 | fat: 11.3g | protein: 32.6g | carbs: 6.4g | net carbs: 5.1g | fiber: 1.3g

Ingredients:

- 4 tablespoons olive oil
- 2 bell peppers, chopped
- 2 red onions, chopped
- 2 teaspoons garlic, minced
- 3 pounds (680 g) chicken wings, boneless
- 4 cups tomato sauce
- 1 tablespoon capers
- 1/2 teaspoon red pepper, crushed
- 1/2 cup Parmesan cheese, preferably freshly grated
- 4 basil sprigs, chopped

Procedure:

1. Firstly, heat the olive oil in a non-stick skillet over a moderate flame.
2. Once hot, sauté the bell peppers and onions until tender and fragrant.
3. Then, stir in the garlic and continue to cook an additional 30 seconds.
4. Now, stir in the chicken wings, tomato sauce, capers, and red pepper; continue to cook for a further 20 minutes or until everything is heated through.
5. Finally, serve garnished with freshly grated Parmesan and basil. Bon appétit!

Italian Parmesan Turkey Fillets

Servings: 10

Preparation Time: 25 minutes

Per Serving: calories: 336 | fat: 12.7g | protein: 47.5g | carbs: 5.2g | net carbs: 5.0g | fiber: 0.2g

Ingredients:

- 4 eggs
- 2 cups sour cream
- 2 teaspoons Italian seasoning blend
- Kosher salt and ground black pepper, to taste
- 1 cup grated Parmesan cheese
- 4 pounds (907 g) turkey fillets

Procedure:

1. Firstly, in a mixing bowl, whisk the eggs until frothy and light.
2. Stir in the sour cream and continue whisking until well combined.
3. Then, in another bowl, mix the Italian seasoning blend with the salt, black pepper, and Parmesan cheese; mix to combine well.

4. Now, dip the turkey fillets into the egg mixture; then, press them into the Parmesan mixture.
5. Finally, cook in the greased frying pan until browned on all sides. Bon appétit!

Dinner

Tasty Cauliflower Soup with Pancetta

Servings: 8

Preparation Time: 50 minutes

Per Serving: Calories: 112 Protein: 10g Fat: 22g Net Carbs: 21g

Ingredients:

- 8 cups chicken broth or vegetable stock
- 30 oz. cauliflower
- 14 oz. cream cheese
- 2 tbsp. Dijon mustard
- 8 oz. butter
- Salt and pepper
- 14 oz. pancetta or bacon, diced
- 2 tbsp. butter, for frying
- 2 teaspoons paprika powder or smoked chili powder
- 6 oz. pecans

Procedure:

1. Firstly, trim the cauliflower and cut it into smaller floret heads.
2. The smaller the florets are, the quicker the soup will be ready.
3. Put aside a handful of the fresh cauliflower and chop into small 1/4 inch bits.

4. Then, sauté the finely chopped cauliflower and pancetta in butter until it is crispy.

5. Add some nuts and the paprika powder at the end.

6. Now, set aside the mixture for serving.

7. Boil the cauliflower until they are soft. Add the cream cheese, mustard, and butter.

8. Stir the soup well, using an immersion blender, to get to the desired consistency.

9. The creamier the soup will become the longer you blend.

10. Salt and pepper the soup to taste.

11. Finally, serve soup in bowls, and top it with the fried pancetta mixture.

Yummy Butter Mayonnaise

Servings: 8

Preparation Time: 45 minutes

Per Serving: 428 Protein: 45g Fat: 4g Net Carbs: 14g

Ingredients:

- 51/3 oz. butter
- 2 eggs yolk
- 2 tbsp. Dijon mustard
- 2 tsp lemon juice
- 1/2 tsp salt
- 2 pinch ground black pepper

Procedure:

1. Firstly, melt the butter in a small saucepan.
2. Pour it into a small pitcher or a jug with a spout and let the butter cool.
3. Then, mix together egg yolks and mustard in a small-sized bowl. Pour the butter in a thin stream while beating it with a hand mixer.
4. Now, leave the sediment that settles at the bottom.

5. Keep beating the mixture until the mayonnaise turns thick and creamy.
6. Add some lemon juice. Season it with salt and black pepper.
7. Finally, serve this immediately.

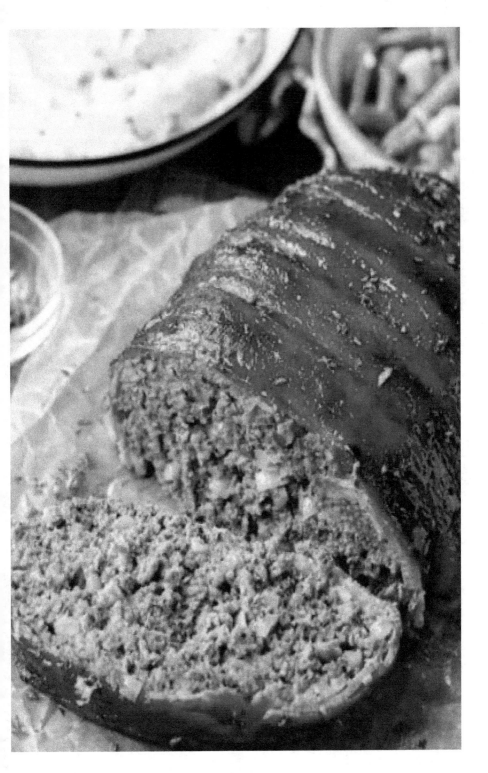

Meatloaf Wrapped in Bacon

Servings: 6

Preparation Time: 25 minutes

Per Serving: Calories: 308 Protein: 21g Fat: 8g Net Carbs: 19g

Ingredients:

- 4 tbsp. butter
- 2 yellow onions, finely chopped
- 50 oz. ground beef or ground lamb/pork
- 1 cup heavy whipping cream
- 1 cup shredded cheese
- 1 egg
- 2 tbsp. dried oregano or dried basil
- 2 tsp salt
- 1 tsp ground black pepper
- 14 oz. sliced bacon
- 3 cups heavy whipping cream, for the gravy

Procedure:

1. Firstly, preheat the oven to 400°F.

2. Fry the onion until it is soft but not overly browned.

3. Mix the ground meat in a bowl with all the other ingredients, minus the bacon.

4. Then, mix it well, but avoid overworking it as you do not want the mixture to become dense.

5. Mold the meat into a loaf shape and place it in a baking dish.

6. Now, wrap the loaf completely in the bacon.

7. Bake the loaf in the middle rack of the oven for about 45 minutes.

8. If you notice that the bacon begins to overcook before the meat is done, cover it with some aluminum foil and lower the heat a bit since you do not want burnt bacon.

9. Save all the juices that have accumulated in the baking dish from the meat and bacon, and use to make the gravy.

10. Mix these juices and the cream in a smaller saucepan for the gravy.

11. Bring it to a boil and lower the heat and let it simmer for 10 to 15 minutes until it has the right consistency and is not lumpy.

12. Finally, serve the meatloaf.

13. Serve with freshly boiled broccoli or some cauliflower with butter, salt, and pepper.

Delicious Keto Salmon with Broccoli Mash

Servings: 10

Preparation Time: 35 minutes

Per Serving: Calories: 156 Protein: 15g Fat: 11g Net Carbs: 5g

Ingredients:

- 3 lbs. salmon
- 1 egg
- 1 yellow onion
- 2 tsp salt
- 1 tsp pepper
- 4 oz. butter, for frying
- Green mash
- 2 lb. broccoli
- 10 oz. butter
- 4 oz. grated parmesan
- Salt and pepper
- Lemon butter:
- 8 oz. butter at room temperature
- 4 tablespoons lemon juice
- Salt and pepper to taste

Procedure:

1. Firstly, preheat the oven to 220° F.
2. Cut the fish into smaller pieces and place them along with the rest of the ingredients for the burger, into a food processor.
3. Blend it for 30 to 45 seconds until you have a rough mixture.
4. Don't mix it too thoroughly as you do not want tough burgers.
5. Then, shape 6 to 8 burgers and fry them for 4 to 5 minutes on each side on a medium heat in a generous amount of butter. Or even oil if you prefer.
6. Keep them warm in the oven.
7. Trim the broccoli and cut it into smaller florets.
8. Now, you can use the stems as well just peel them and chop it into small pieces.
9. Bring a pot of salted water to a boil and add the broccoli to this.
10. Cook it for a few minutes until it is soft, but not until all the texture is gone.
11. Drain and discard the water used for boiling.
12. Use an immersion blender or even a food processor to mix the broccoli with the butter and the parmesan cheese.
13. Season the broccoli mash to taste with salt and pepper.
14. Make the lemon butter by mixing room temperature butter with lemon juice, salt and pepper into a small bowl using electric beaters.
15. Finally, serve the warm burgers with the side of green broccoli mash and a melting dollop of fresh lemon butter on top of the burger.

Tempting Oven Baked Sausage and Vegetables

Servings: 4

Preparation Time: 35 minutes

Per Serving: Calories: 176 Protein: 31g Fat: 12g Net Carbs: 10g

Ingredients:

- 2 oz. butter, for greasing the baking dish
- 2 small zucchini
- 4 yellow onions
- 6 garlic cloves
- 51/3 oz. tomatoes
- 14 oz. fresh mozzarella
- Sea salt
- Black pepper
- 2 tbsp. dried basil
- Olive oil
- 2 lb. sausages in links, in links

For Servings:

- 1 cup mayonnaise

Procedure:

1. Firstly, preheat the oven to 400°F. Grease the baking dish with butter.
2. Divide the zucchini into bite-sized pieces.
3. Peel and cut the onion into wedges.
4. Slice or chop the garlic.
5. Then, place zucchini, onions, garlic, and tomatoes in the baking dish.
6. Dice the cheese and place among the vegetables.
7. Season with salt, pepper and basil.
8. Sprinkle olive oil over the vegetables, and top with sausage.
9. Now, bake until the sausages are thoroughly cooked and the vegetables are browned.
10. Finally, serve with a dollop of mayonnaise.

Enjoyable Herbs Pork Chops

Servings: 8

Preparation Time: 30 minutes

Per Serving: Calories: 333 Protein: 31g Fat: 23g Net Carbs: 0g

Ingredients:

- 4 Tablespoons Butter + More for Coating
- 8 Pork Chops, Boneless
- 4 Tablespoons Italian Leaf Parsley Chopped
- Sea Salt & Black Pepper to Taste
- 4 Tablespoons Italian Seasoning
- 4 Tablespoons Olive Oil

Procedure:

1. Firstly, start by heating your oven to 350 and coat a baking dish with butter.
2. Season your pork chops, and then top with fresh parsley, drizzling with olive oil and a half a tablespoon of butter each to bake.
3. Then, bake for twenty to twenty-five minutes.

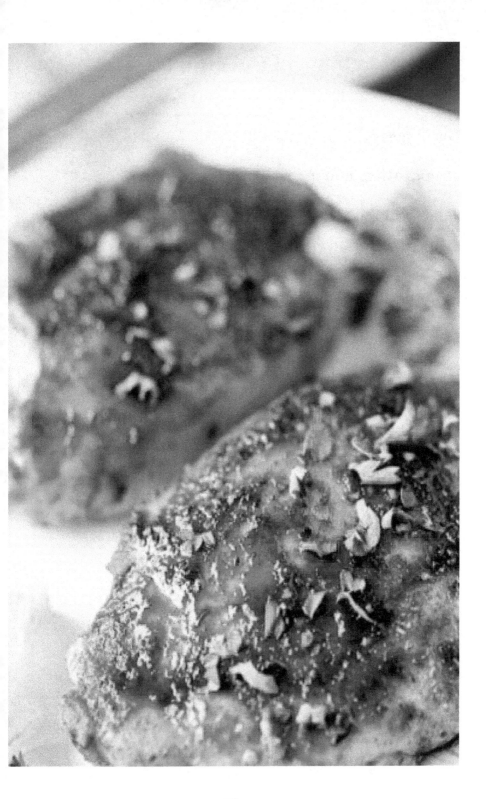

Delightful Coconut Chicken

Servings: 8

Preparation Time: 40 minutes

Per Serving: Calories: 382 Protein: 23g Fat: 31g Net Carbs: 4g

Ingredients:

- 2 Teaspoon Ground Cumin
- 2 Teaspoon Ground Coriander
- 1/2 Cup Cilantro, Fresh & Chopped
- 2 Cups Coconut Milk
- 2 Tablespoons Curry Powder
- 4 Tablespoons Olive Oil
- 1 Cup Sweet Onion, Chopped
- 8 Chicken Breasts, 4 Ounces Each & Cut into 2 Inch Chunks

Procedure:

1. Firstly, get out a saucepan, adding in your oil and heating it over medium-high heat.
2. Sauté your chicken until it's almost completely cooked, which will take roughly ten minutes.
3. Then, add in your onion, cooking for another three minutes.

4. Whisk your curry powder, coconut milk, coriander and cumin together.

5. Now, pour the sauce into your pan, bringing it to a boil with your chicken.

6. Reduce the heat, and let it simmer for ten minutes.

7. Finally, serve topped with cilantro.

Tasty Double Cheese Stuffed Venison

Servings: 4

Preparation Time: 35 minutes

Per Serving: calories: 196 | fat: 11.9g | protein: 25.1g | carbs: 2.1g | net carbs: 1.6g | fiber: 0.5g

Ingredients:

- 1 pounds (907 g) venison tenderloin
- 1 garlic cloves, minced
- 1 tablespoon chopped almonds
- 1/2 cup Gorgonzola cheese
- 1/4 cup Feta cheese
- 1/2 teaspoon chopped onion
- 1/2 teaspoon salt

Procedure:

1. Firstly, preheat your grill to medium.
2. Slice the tenderloin lengthwise to make a pocket for the filling.
3. Combine the rest of the ingredients in a bowl.
4. Then, stuff the tenderloin with the filling.
5. Now, shut the meat with skewers and grill for as long as it takes to reach your desired density.

Veal with Ham and Sauerkraut

Servings: 8

Preparation Time: 1 hour 10 minutes

Per Serving: calories: 431 | fat: 26.9g | protein: 28.6g | carbs: 10.1g | net carbs: 5.9g | fiber: 4.2g

Ingredients:

- 2 pounds (454 g) veal, cut into cubes
- 16 ounces (510 g) sauerkraut, rinsed and drained
- Salt and black pepper, to taste
- 1 cup ham, chopped
- 1 onion, chopped
- 4 garlic cloves, minced
- 2 tablespoons butter
- 1 cup Parmesan cheese, grated
- 1 cup sour cream

Procedure:

1. Firstly, heat a pot with the butter over medium heat, add in the onion, and cook for 3 minutes.
2. Stir in garlic, and cook for 1 minute.

3. Then, place in the veal and ham, and cook until slightly browned.
4. Now, place in the sauerkraut, and cook until the meat becomes tender, about 30 minutes.
5. Stir in sour cream, pepper, and salt.
6. Finally, top with Parmesan cheese and bake for 20 minutes at 350°F (180°C).

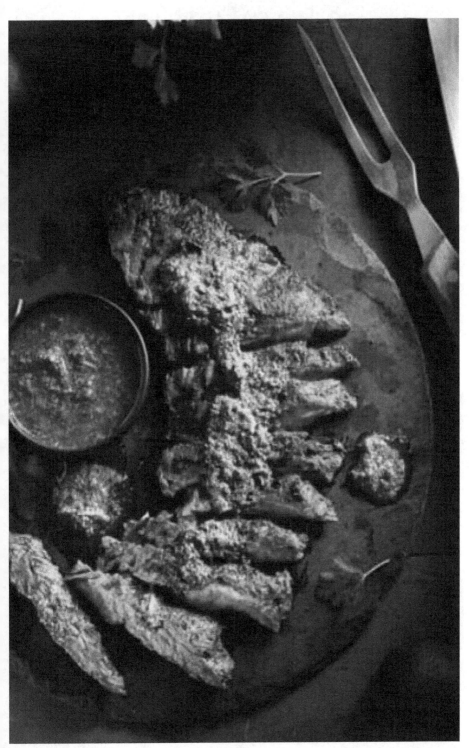

Balsamic Skirt Steak

Servings: 12

Preparation Time: 10 minutes

Per Serving: calories: 355 | fat: 25.1g | protein: 30.9g | carbs: 0g | net carbs: 0g | fiber: 0g

Ingredients:

- 1/2 cup balsamic vinegar (no sugar added)
- 4 tablespoons extra-virgin olive oil
- tablespoons fresh chopped parsley
- teaspoons minced garlic
- 2 teaspoons kosher salt
- 1/2 teaspoon ground black pepper
- pounds (907 g) skirt steak, trimmed of fat

Procedure:

1. Firstly, in a medium-sized bowl, whisk together the vinegar, olive oil, parsley, garlic, salt, and pepper.
2. Add the skirt steak and flip to ensure that the entire surface is covered in marinade.
3. Cover with plastic wrap and marinate in the refrigerator for at least 2 hours, or up to 24 hours.

4. Then, take the bowl out of the refrigerator and let the steak and marinade come to room temperature.

5. Meanwhile, preheat a grill to high heat.

6. Remove the steak from the marinade (reserve the marinade) and place on the grill over direct high heat.

7. Grill for 3 minutes per side for medium (recommended) or 5 minutes per side for well-done.

8. Now, remove the steak from the grill when the desired doneness is reached and let rest for 10 minutes before slicing.

9. Meanwhile, place the reserved marinade in the microwave and cook on high for 3 minutes, or until boiling.

10. Stir and set aside; you will use the boiled marinade as a sauce for the steak.

11. Slice the steak, being sure to cut against the grain for best results.

12. Finally, serve with the sauce.

Easy Beef Chunk Chili Con Carne

Servings: 12

Preparation Time: 2 hours 20 minutes

Per Serving: calories: 364 | fat: 26.9g | protein: 28.9g | carbs: 3.6g | net carbs: 2.0g | fiber: 1.6g

Ingredients:

- 4 pounds (907 g) boneless beef chuck, trimmed and cut into 1-inch cubes
- 1 teaspoon kosher salt
- 1 teaspoon ground black pepper
- 4 tablespoons avocado oil or other light-tasting oil
- 2 cups chopped yellow onions
- 2 tablespoons minced garlic
- 6 cups beef broth, store-bought or homemade
- 2 tablespoons chili powder
- 4 teaspoons ground cumin
- 2 teaspoons cayenne pepper
- 2 teaspoons dried oregano leaves
- 2 teaspoons ground coriander
- 1/2 teaspoon ground cinnamon

- 1/2 cup canned chipotles in adobo sauce
- 1 tablespoon apple cider vinegar
- 2 tablespoons coconut flour

Procedure:

1. Firstly, season the beef with the salt and pepper.
2. Heat the oil in a large heavy-bottomed saucepan (make sure it has a lid) or a 4- or 6-quart Dutch oven over medium-high heat.
3. Add the beef and brown on all sides, about 4 minutes. Remove the meat and set aside.
4. Add the onions and garlic to the pan and cook for 5 minutes, or until browned and translucent.
5. Then, add the meat back to the pan along with the broth, spices, and chipotles.
6. Simmer, covered, until the meat is tender, about 2 hours.
7. Now, stir in the vinegar.
8. Remove about ¼ cup of the sauce to a small bowl.
9. Whisk the coconut flour into the bowl of sauce, then add the sauce back to the pot and stir well.
10. Simmer, uncovered, for 5 more minutes, until the sauce has thickened.
11. Finally, taste and season with more salt and pepper, if desired.

Flavorful Pepperoni and Beef Pizza Meatloaf

Servings: 4

Preparation Time: 1 hour 10 minutes

Per Serving: calories: 440 | fat: 30.9g | protein: 32.8g | carbs: 3.4g | net carbs: 2.4g | fiber: 1.0g

Ingredients:

- 1 pound (907 g) ground beef (80/20)
- ⅓ cup superfine blanched almond flour
- 1/8 cup grated Parmesan cheese
- 1/2 tablespoon dried parsley
- 1/2 tablespoon dried onion flakes
- 1/2 teaspoon kosher salt
- 1/4 teaspoon dried oregano leaves
- 1/4 teaspoon garlic powder
- 1/4 teaspoon ground black pepper
- 1 large eggs
- 1/2 cup marinara sauce, store-bought or homemade, plus more for serving if desired
- 1 cup shredded whole-milk Mozzarella cheese
- 2 ounces (113 g) thinly sliced pepperoni
- Chopped fresh parsley, for garnish (optional)

Procedure:

1. Firstly, preheat the oven to 375°F (190°C). Line a 9 by 5-inch loaf pan with foil, leaving 2 inches of foil folded over the outside edges of the pan.
2. The extra foil will make it easier to lift the cooked meatloaf out of the pan.
3. Place the ground beef, almond flour, Parmesan cheese, parsley, onion flakes, salt, oregano, garlic powder, pepper, and eggs in a large bowl and mix well by hand until the texture is uniform.
4. Then, press the meatloaf mixture into the prepared loaf pan and flatten it out.
5. Spoon the marinara evenly over the top and then sprinkle with the Mozzarella cheese.
6. Layer the pepperoni slices on top.
7. Bake, uncovered, for 1 hour, or until a meat thermometer inserted in the center reads 165°F (74°C).
8. Now, remove the meatloaf from the oven and let cool for at least 10 minutes in the pan to allow it to firm up before slicing.
9. Carefully remove the meatloaf from the pan using the foil as handles.
10. Place on a cutting board and remove the foil.
11. Finally, you can then cut it into slices and serve on individual plates, or, to dress it up a bit, spread some warm marinara sauce on the bottom of a serving platter, then place the loaf on top of the sauce and garnish with fresh parsley, as shown.

Dessert

Tasty Cardamom Butter

Servings: 12

Preparation Time: 10 minutes

Per Serving: 3.5 g of net Carbs 8.8 g of protein 14 g oFat 1.7 g o
Fiber 176.6 of Cal

Ingredients:

- 1 cup blanched almond flour
- 1/2 tsp baking powder (straight phosphate, double effect)
- 1 tsp salt
- 20 Tbsp unsalted butter
- 1 cup sucralose sweetener (sugar substitute)
- 2 large egg (whole)
- 2 Tbsp tap water
- 2 tsp vanilla extract
- 3/4 tsp ground cardamom
- 8 2/3 Servings:, flour mixture

Procedure:

1. First, use the flour mixture (or the gluten-free version) for this
   . To make 12 Serving , you need 1 ½ cups of the mix.
2. If you change the size of the portion to increase or decrease it,
   you must adjust it accordingly.
3. Each serving of the baking blend represents ⅓ cup.
4. Preheat the oven to 350° F.
5. Then, cover 2 baking sheets with parchment paper; put aside.
6. In a medium bowl, add 1 ½ cup baking mixture, ½ cup almond
   flour, baking powder, and salt. In a large bowl, blend butter and
   sugar substitute; cream until soft and fluffy with an electric
   mixer at high speed.
7. Now, add the egg, sugar, vanilla, and cardamom; beat until
   smooth at medium speed; scrape the bowl sides if necessary
   (the mixture can appear watery).
8. Add the flour mixture; blend until the dough is gathered.
9. Cut the dough in half and then again in half. Create 6 equal
   balls out of every quarter of the dough piece. Place on baking
   sheet 12 mixture.
10. Gently squeeze each with the teeth of a grid fork (optional);
    cook about 10 min on the light brown edge.
11. Or put it 30 min in the refrigerator and spread it over the
    parchment; cut the shapes and cook.
12. To cool them, move cookies to a wire rack. Store up to 1 week in
    an airtight container.
13. Finally, makes 2 cookies for each serving.

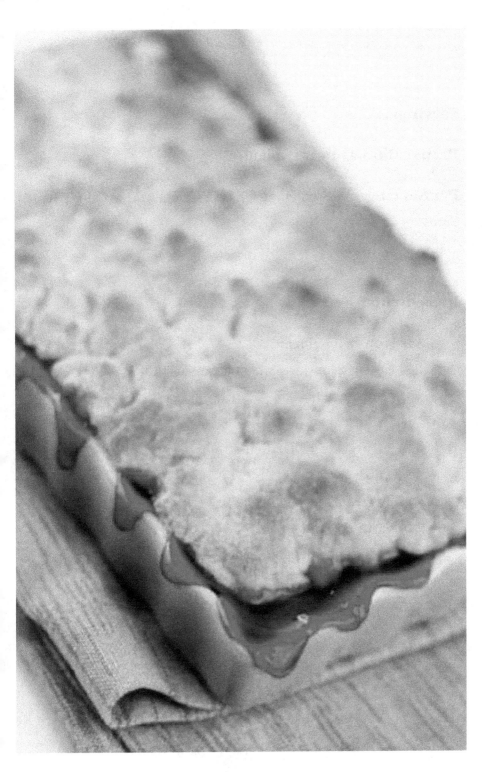

Cherry Cobbler

Servings: 4

Preparation Time: 30 minutes

Per Serving: 7.4 g protein 12.9 g fat 2.5 g fiber 191.2 Cal 11 g net Carbs

Ingredients:

- 1/8 cup, half walnuts
- ¼ cup sucralose sweetener (sugar substitute)
- 3/4 cinnamon tsp
- 1/8 tsp salt
- 1.1/2 Tbsp unsalted butter bar
- 1/3 cup heavy cream
- 1 sour cream Tbsp (cultivated)
- 1/2 large egg (whole)
- 1.1/2 cups, no Sweet bites cherries
- 1/8 tsp pure almond extract
- 1 ¼ Servings:, flour mixture

Procedure:

For the cookies:

1. Firstly, mix baking mix, nuts, 2 Tbsp sugar substitute, ½ tsp cinnamon, and salt in a food processor until it is moderately ground.
2. Add the butter and squeeze until mixture looks like a full meal.
3. Then, beat the heavy cream, sour cream, and an egg in a cup or bowl to measure liquids.
4. Pour into a food processor and press until everything is well mixed.
5. Remove the dough and tap on a flat disc.
6. Now, cover with plastic wrap and allow to cool for 1 to 2 hours.
7. For the filling: Preheat the oven to 400° F.
8. Mix the cherries in a medium bowl with ⅓ cup sugar substitute, almond extract, and ¼ tsp cinnamon.
9. Pour the filling into an 8-inch square or round baking dish. Divide the dough into 8 pieces and pat it on discs about 3 wide.
10. Alternate the cookies on the filling and bake for 35 to 40 min, until the cookies are golden and cooked and the fruit bubbles are soft.
11. Finally, serve with fresh whipped cream (optional).

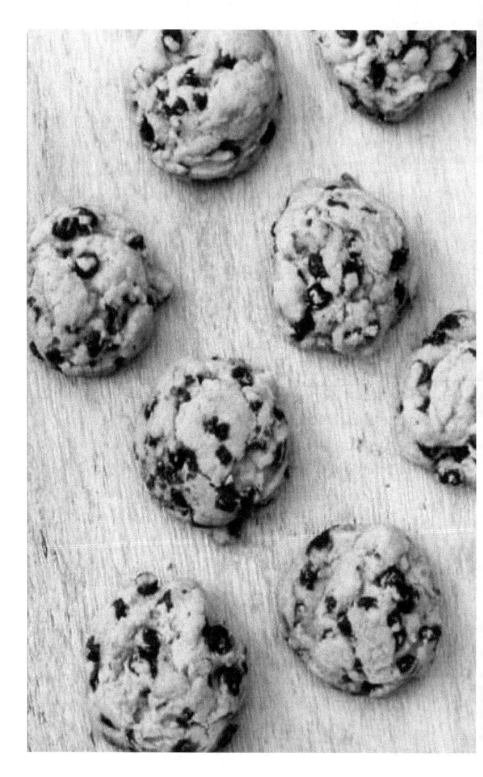

Chocolate Chip Cookies

Servings: 12

Preparation Time: 20 minutes

Per Serving: 2 g net Carbs 3.8 g protein 7.1 g fat 1.4 g fiber 86.7 Cal

Ingredients:

- 2 tsp baking powder
- 1 tsp salt
- 2 cups butter (salted)
- 2 cups sucralose sweetener (sugar substitute)
- 4 tsp vanilla extract
- 4 large eggs (whole)
- 8 g sugar-free Chocolate Chips
- 12 Servings: flour mixture

Procedure:

1. Firstly, preheat the oven to 375° F.
2. Combine all dry ingredients in a small bowl, set aside.
3. Mix melted butter, sugar substitute, and vanilla on medium speed with an electric mixer until everything is well combined.
4. Add eggs 1 by 1 and mix well after each addition.

5. Then, gradually add the mixture of dry ingredients and beat until well blended.

6. Thoroughly mix the chocolate chips with a wooden spoon or spatula (4 oz or about 2/3 of a cup).

7. A spoon of rounded tsp cookie dough on a baking sheet covered with a spray of non-stick vegetable oil.

8. Now. carefully flatten the cookies by squeezing them with your hand or with a spatula.

9. Finally, make for 10 to 12 min or until light brown. Remove from the baking sheet and place cookies on a cooling rack.

Delectable Frozen Chocolate Pudding Pops

Servings: 2

Preparation Time: 5 minutes

Per Serving: 2 g net Carbs 4.9 g protein 18.9 g fat 1.5 g fiber 196.9 Cal

Ingredients:

- 2 each, generous dark chocolate smoothie
- 3/4 cup heavy cream, liquid
- 2 Tbsp cocoa powder
- 2 Tbsp erythritol
- 1/2 tsp xanthan gum

Procedure:

1. First, you need silicone molds for this .
2. Put all the ingredients in a high power mixer and mix about half at maximum speed for about 2 min the mixture should be a little frothy and well combined.
3. Then, pour mixture into silicone molds and place in the freezer until it is firm, according to the instructions of the silicone mold.
4. Now, use within 2 weeks of freezing.

Crockpot Apple Pudding Cake

Servings: 5

Preparation Time: 20 minutes

Per Serving: Cal 405 Fat 9 g Saturated fat 3 g Carbs 79 g Fiber 2 g
Sugar 63 g Protein 3 g

Ingredient:

- 1/2 cup milk
- 1.1/2 tsp of baking soda
- 1/4 cup cold butter
- cup orange juice
- 1/4 cup honey or brown sugar
- 1/2 tsp cinnamon

Procedure:

1. Firstly, combine flour, 2/3 cup sugar, baking powder, and salt. Cut the butter until you have thick crumbs in the mixture.
2. Remove the milk from the crumbs until it becomes moist.
3. Then, grease the bottom and sides of a 4 or 5-liter slow cooker. Place the dough at the bottom of the pot and spread it evenly.
4. Now, heat the orange juice, honey, butter, remaining sugar and cinnamon in a medium pan.

5. Decorate the apples.

6. Place the jar opening with a clean cloth, place the lid.

7. Prevents condensation on the cover from reaching the pot.

8. Finally, place the pan on top and cook until apples are tender for 2 to 3 hours.

Enticing Chocolate Caramel Monkey Bread

Servings: 12

Preparation Time: 10 minutes

Per Serving: Cal 337k saturated fat 16g Carbs 44g Fiber 1g Sugar 12g Protein 5g

Ingredients:

- 2 Tbsp sugar
- 1/2 tsp ground cinnamon
- 40 candies coated with milk chocolate
- 30 oz whey cookies
- chocolate sauce to include (optional
- caramel sauce to cover (optional)

Procedure:

1. Firstly, mix sugar and cinnamon and set aside.
2. Fill a jar with parchment paper, cover to the bottom.
3. Then, wrap 1 buttermilk cookie dough around a chocolate candy to completely cover the candy and close the seam.
4. Place the candy wrapped in cookies at the bottom of the jar, start in the middle of the pot and continue on the side.

5. Now, continue to wrap the candies and place them in the slow cooker, leaving about ½ inch between each.
6. Repeat these steps with sweets wrapped in the second layer of cookies.
7. Sprinkle the rest of the sugar and cinnamon mixture over the dough.
8. Cover the pan and cook for 1 hour 30 min.
9. After cooking, remove the cover and allow it to cool slightly.
10. Use the edges of the parchment paper to lift the monkey bread from the jar and move it onto a wire rack. Let cool for at least 10-15 min
11. Cut off the excess baking paper around the edge when you're ready to serve.
12. Finally, place the monkey bread in a shallow pan or bowl and sprinkle with chocolate sauce and caramel sauce.

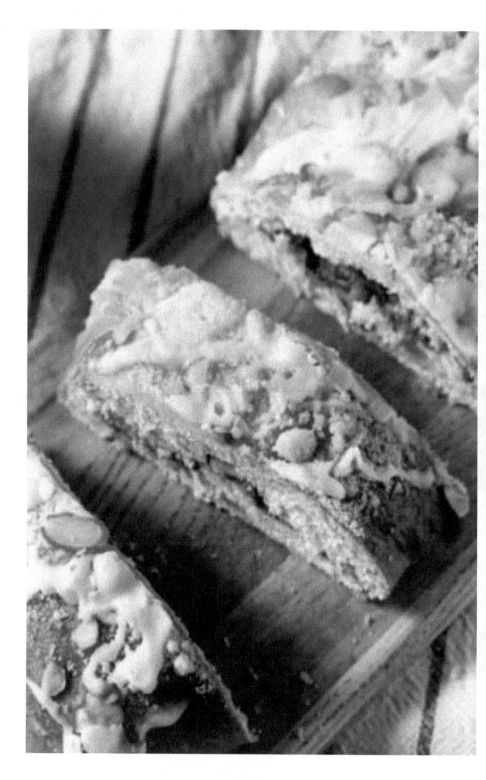

Coffee Cake

Servings: 6

Preparation Time: 10 minutes

Per Serving: Cal 411, Carbs 56 g, Protein 6g, Fat 19 g Saturated Fat 3g, Fiber 2g, Sugar 33 g

Ingredients:

- 1 cups all-purpose flour
- ¾ cups packed brown sugar
- cups almond milk
- 2/3 cups vegetable oil
- 1 tsp of baking soda
- 1/2 tsp ground cinnamon
- 1/4 tsp of baking soda
- 1/2 tsp white vinegar
- 1/2 tsp salt
- 1 egg
- 1/4 cup optional chopped nuts

Procedure:

1. First, beat flour, brown sugar, and salt in a large bowl.
2. Add the oil until it is crumbly.
3. Mix baking powder, baking powder, and cinnamon with a wooden spoon or spatula in the flour mixture.
4. Place the milk, oil, eggs, and vinegar in a measuring cup and mix until the eggs are crushed, add them to the flour mixture and stir until they are combined (the dough may be slightly lumpy).
5. Then, spray a 5-7Q non-stick cooking spray or a line with a slow cooking spray.
6. Pour into the pot with the dough.
7. Sprinkle nuts over the cake dough at the end.
8. Place a large paper towel over the insert and place the lid on it.
9. Now, cook over high heat for 1 ½ to 2 ½ hours or until a toothpick is used to clean the edges.
10. The middle is perhaps a little poorly done at the top.
11. Serve hot directly from the slow cooker or keep up to 3 days in an airtight container.
12. Use the slow cooker liner to serve effectively.
13. You can lift the whole box, peel it off, and help the cake this way.
14. Finally, use a 9 x 13-inch pan sprayed with non-stick cooking oil in a conventional oven and bake for about 35 to 45 min

Yummy Mocha Mousse

Servings: 12

Preparation Time: 10 minutes

Per Serving: calories: 126 | fat: 11.9g | protein: 0g | carbs: 3.1g | net carbs: 2.0g | fiber: 1.1g

Ingredients:

- 2 (13.5-ounce / 383-g) can coconut cream, chilled overnight
- 6 tablespoons granulated erythritol–monk fruit blend; less sweet: 2 tablespoons
- tablespoons unsweetened cocoa powder, plus more for dusting
- 2 teaspoons instant espresso powder
- 1/2 teaspoon salt

Procedure:

1. Firstly, put the large metal bowl in the freezer to chill for at least 1 hour.
2. Then, in the chilled large bowl, using an electric mixer on high, combine the coconut cream (adding it by the spoonful and reserving the water that has separated), erythritol–monk fruit blend, the cocoa powder, espresso powder, and salt and beat for

3 to 5 minutes, until stiff peaks form, stopping and scraping the bowl once or twice, as needed.

3. If the consistency is too thick, add the reserved water from the coconut cream 1 tablespoon at a time to thin.

4. Now, serve immediately in a cold glass, dusted with cocoa powder.

5. Finally, store leftovers in an airtight container for up to 5 days in the refrigerator.

Cinnamon Cream Cheese Mousse

Servings: 4

Preparation Time: 15 minutes

Per Serving: calories: 274 | fat: 28.9g | protein: 3.1g | carbs: 3.1g | net carbs: 1.9g | fiber: 1.2g

Ingredients:

- 2 ounces (57 g) full-fat cream cheese, at room temperature
- 2 cups heavy whipping cream, divided
- 1/2 cup granulated erythritol–monk fruit blend; less sweet: 2 tablespoons
- 1/4 teaspoon vanilla extract
- 1/4 teaspoon salt
- 1 cup finely milled almond flour
- 1/4 cup coconut flour
- 1/4 cup granulated erythritol–monk fruit blend
- 1/2 teaspoon ground cinnamon
- 1/8 teaspoon sea salt
- 2 tablespoons (½ stick) cold unsalted butter, thinly sliced

Procedure:

1. Firstly, put the large metal bowl in the freezer to chill for at least 5 minutes.

2. In the large chilled bowl, using an electric mixer on medium high, mix the cream cheese and ¼ cup of heavy cream until well combined.

3. Then, add the erythritol–monk fruit blend, vanilla, and salt and mix until just combined.

4. Add the remaining 1¼ cups of heavy cream and beat on high for about 3 minutes, until stiff peaks form, stopping and scraping the bowl once or twice, as needed.

5. Now, refrigerate for at least 1 hour and up to overnight before serving.

6. In the small bowl, combine the almond flour, coconut flour, erythritol–monk fruit blend, cinnamon, and salt.

7. Add the sliced butter and combine using a fork until the mixture resembles coarse crumbs.

8. Finally, set aside until ready to serve.

9. Serve the mousse in short glasses or small mason jars topped with the crumble.

10. Store leftovers in an airtight container for up to 5 days in the refrigerator.

Blueberry and Strawberry

Servings: 5

Preparation Time: 50 minutes

Per Serving: calories: 440 | fat: 41.9g | protein: 8.0g | carbs: 8.9g | net carbs: 7.0g | fiber: 1.9g

Ingredients:

- 2 tablespoons unsalted butter, at room temperature, plus more for greasing
- 1cups finely milled almond flour, sifted
- 1/2 teaspoon baking powder
- 1/8 teaspoon salt
- ¾ cup granulated erythritol–monk fruit blend; less sweet: ½ cup
- 2 ounces (113 g) full-fat cream cheese, at room temperature
- 1 teaspoon vanilla extract
- 2 large eggs, at room temperature
- 1/2 cup fresh or frozen blueberries
- 2 ounces (227 g) fresh or frozen strawberries, thinly sliced
- 1 tablespoons granulated erythritol–monk fruit blend; less sweet: 1 tablespoon
- 1/4 tablespoon freshly squeezed lemon juice
- 1 cup heavy whipping cream

- 2 ounces (227 g) full-fat cream cheese, at room temperature
- 1/8 cup granulated erythritol–monk fruit blend; less sweet: 2 tablespoons
- 1/2 teaspoon vanilla extract

Procedure:

1. Firstly, preheat the oven to 350°F (180°C).
2. Grease the loaf pan with butter, line with parchment paper, and set aside.
3. In a medium bowl, combine the almond flour, baking powder, and salt. Set aside.
4. In a large bowl, using an electric mixer on high, cream the butter with the erythritol–monk fruit blend for 2 to 3 minutes, stopping and scraping the bowl once or twice, as needed, until the mixture is light and fluffy and well incorporated.
5. Add the cream cheese and vanilla and mix well.
6. Then, add the eggs, one at a time, making sure to mix well after each addition.
7. Add the dry ingredients to the wet ingredients and mix well until the batter is fully combined.
8. Scrape the batter into the prepared loaf pan.
9. Now, bake for 30 to 40 minutes, until golden brown on top and a toothpick inserted into the center comes out clean.
10. Remove from the oven and set aside to cool before slicing.
11. While the cake is baking, in another large bowl, combine the blueberries, strawberries, erythritol–monk fruit blend, and lemon juice.
12. Toss until fully coated and set aside.

13. In a third large bowl, using an electric mixer on high, whip the heavy cream for 3 to 5 minutes, until stiff peaks form, stopping and scraping the bowl once or twice, as needed.

14. In another medium bowl, using an electric mixer on medium high, beat the cream cheese and erythritol–monk fruit blend for 1 to 2 minutes, until smooth and creamy, then stir in the vanilla.

15. Gently fold the whipped cream into the cream cheese mixture until well combined.

16. Assemble the trifle by breaking the slices of the cake into pieces that fit into the bottom of the trifle dish.

17. Add one-third of the berry mixture, followed by one-third of the whipped cream.

18. Alternate the layers two more times, ending with the whipped cream on top.

19. Finally, store leftovers covered in an airtight container for up to 3 days in the refrigerator.

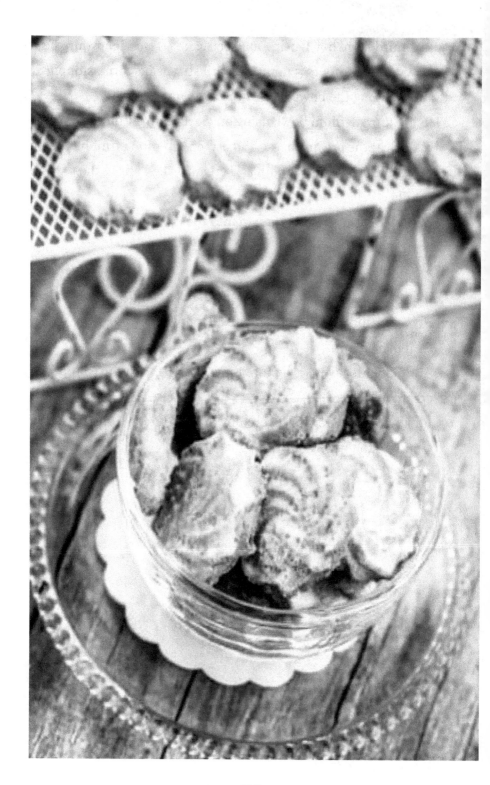

Butter Cookies

Servings: 12

Preparation Time: 30 minutes

Per Serving: calories: 235 | fat: 21.9g | protein: 6.0g | carbs: 6.0g | net carbs: 4.0g | fiber: 2.0g

Ingredients:

- 1/2 cup granulated erythritol–monk fruit blend
- tablespoons (1 stick) unsalted butter, at room temperature
- 1/2 teaspoon vanilla extract
- 2 large eggs, at room temperature
- 1/4 cup full-fat sour cream
- 2 cup finely milled almond flour, sifted
  - teaspoons baking powder
- 1/8 teaspoon sea salt
- 1 cup confectioners' erythritol–monk fruit blend
- 1/4 cup full-fat sour cream
- 1/4 teaspoon vanilla extract

Procedure:

1. Firstly, preheat the oven to 350°F (180°C).
2. Line the baking sheet with parchment paper and set aside.
3. In the medium bowl, using an electric mixer on high, combine the granulated erythritol–monk fruit blend, butter, and vanilla for 1 to 2 minutes, until light and fluffy, stopping and scraping the bowl once or twice, as needed.
4. Add the eggs, one at a time, to the medium bowl, then add the sour cream. Mix until well incorporated.
5. Then, next add the almond flour, baking powder, and salt and mix until just combined.
6. Put the dough in the refrigerator and chill for 30 minutes.
7. Drop the dough in tablespoons on the prepared baking sheet evenly spaced about 1 inch apart.
8. Bake the cookies for 15 to 20 minutes, until lightly browned around the edges.
9. Now, transfer the cookies to a cooling rack to fully cool, 15 to 20 minutes.
10. In the small bowl, combine the confectioners' erythritol–monk fruit blend, sour cream, and vanilla.
11. Once the cookies are fully cooled, using a spoon or pastry bag, drizzle the icing on top to serve.
12. Finally, store leftovers in the refrigerator for up to 5 days or freeze for up to 3 weeks.

Pleasant Cinnamon Gingerbread

Servings: 12

Preparation Time: 30 minutes

Per Serving: calories: 107 | fat: 9.0g | protein: 3.0g | carbs: 5.0g | net carbs: 3.0g | fiber: 2.0g

Ingredients:

- 1 cup brown or golden erythritol–monk fruit blend; less sweet: 1¼ cups
- 1.1/2 large eggs
- tablespoons (½ stick) unsalted butter, at room temperature
- 1/2 tablespoon molasses or 1 teaspoon molasses extract (optional)
- 1/2 teaspoon vanilla extract
- 2 tablespoons ground cinnamon
- 1.1/2 tablespoons ground ginger
- ½ teaspoon ground nutmeg
- 1/8 teaspoon ground cloves
- 1.1/2 cups finely milled almond flour
- 1 tablespoon psyllium husk powder
- 1 teaspoons baking powder

- 1/8 teaspoon salt
- 1/8 cup confectioners' erythritol–monk fruit blend
- 1/2 tablespoon heavy whipping cream

Procedure:

1. Firstly, preheat the oven to 325°F (163°C).
2. Line the baking sheet with parchment paper and set aside.
3. In the large bowl, using an electric mixer on high, beat the brown erythritol–monk fruit blend, eggs, butter, molasses (if using), and vanilla until fully incorporated, stopping and scraping the bowl once or twice, as needed.
4. Then, add the cinnamon, ginger, nutmeg, and cloves to the mixture and stir to combine.
5. Add the almond flour, psyllium powder, baking powder, and salt and beat on medium high until well incorporated.
6. Now, place the dough between two sheets of parchment paper and flatten with a rolling pin.
7. Chill the dough in the refrigerator for 30 minutes.
8. Using a small cookie cutter or small-mouthed glass jar, cut the dough into cookies and place them about 1 inch apart, evenly spaced, on the prepared baking sheet.
9. Bake for 12 to 15 minutes, until golden brown.
10. Allow them to cool completely on the cooling rack, 15 to 20 minutes.
11. In the small bowl, combine the confectioners' erythritol–monk fruit blend with the heavy cream 1 teaspoon at a time to make the icing.
12. The icing should have a runny consistency.

13. Decorate the cooled cookies using either a pastry bag for fine detail or drizzle the icing on using a fork for a quick, fuss-free decorated cookie.
14. Finally, store leftovers in an airtight container in the refrigerator for up to 5 days or freeze for up to 3 weeks.

CPSIA information can be obtained
at www.ICGtesting.com
Printed in the USA
BVHW091521100621
609271BV00004B/810

9 781802 996944